The Daily Gratitude Journal for Men

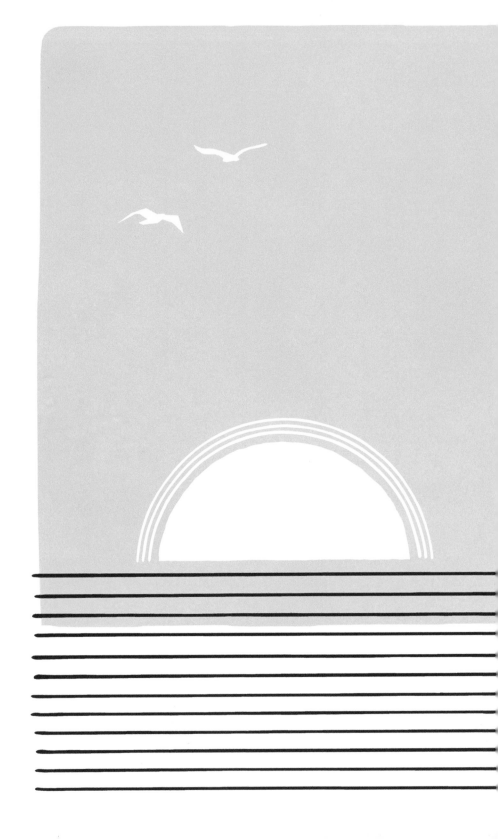

THE *Daily* GRATITUDE JOURNAL FOR MEN

● 90 Days of Mindfulness
and Reflection

Dean Bokhari

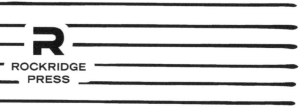

ROCKRIDGE
PRESS

Interior and Cover Designer: Gabe Nansen
Art Producer: Tom Hood
Editor: Jed Bickman

ISBN: 978-1-64876-001-3

R0

CONTENTS

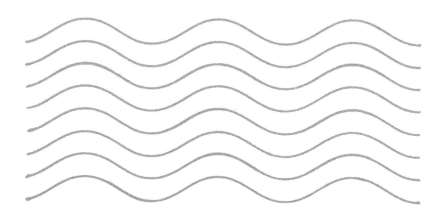

This Journal Belongs To:

_____

INTRODUCTION

Congratulations!

By starting a gratitude journal, you're starting something that could totally transform your life—that's what it's done for me.

As a man, it isn't always easy to talk about your feelings. You're typically conditioned to think you need to avoid showing your emotions and to appear strong at all times. And for a long time, that's exactly how I operated: I buried my emotions and pretended that I was fine. But I wasn't fine. I was far from fine. Truth be told, I felt empty inside.

Then one day, I read about the power of journaling and how it's changed the lives of some of history's most influential men, including:

Benjamin Franklin   Charles Darwin
Leonardo da Vinci   Ernest Hemingway
Jim Rohn   Pablo Picasso

These men were pioneers and prolific creators; they were leaders and life-long learners, and some of the men that many look up to. Well, I wanted to be a great man, too. So, I bought a notebook and started journaling the very same day.

But what was I supposed to write about? How many drinks I had the night before? All the cool things I wanted to do? My goals? These were good ideas, but I wanted to journal about something deeper.

After some trial and error, I realized something incredible: I felt so much better when I wrote about the things I was grateful for in life. I somehow felt lighter and stronger at the same time. I felt more confident and content with my place in the world. I felt calmer. I became less likely to fly off the handle and more likely to respond to people and situations in an emotionally intelligent way. I became less likely to get upset when things didn't go my way, and more likely to feel a deep sense of gratitude for all of the things that actually did go my way. All of these things happened thanks to journaling.

The habit of gratitude journaling has given me the personal power I've been searching for my entire adult life. It's helped me realize that being a man is not about burying your emotions, it's about embracing the full spectrum of your emotions—and gratitude is part of that.

More than a decade has passed since I picked up my first notebook and began gratitude journaling, and I've kept up the habit ever since.

These days, as someone who writes and speaks about motivation and personal development, gratitude journaling is one of the tools I find myself recommending to people over and over again. This tool can help you become the best version of yourself:

- If you've got anger-problems, gratitude journaling helps you find some calm in chaotic situations.

- If you're never satisfied, gratitude journaling helps you uncover all the things you can be genuinely thankful for.

- If you find it difficult to tap into a sense of awareness and intention about the direction your life is headed in, gratitude journaling helps with that, too.

What Makes This Journal *Different?*

A simple framework to guide you, based on the different components of gratitude, which include (1) Awareness, (2) Intention, and (3) Living in Gratitude. Having a structured layout like this simplifies the entire journaling process—no need to stare at a blank page worrying about what to write.

Complementary content such as breath-work reminders, space to draw or jot down thoughts, and sidebars filled with inspiring insights and ideas—all included within your journal.

Inspiring coaching tips to make gratitude journaling a habit. Practicing gratitude isn't always easy. I will be there to help you bring the game-changing power of gratitude into your daily life with this journal.

Maybe this journal was gifted to you. Maybe you went out and found it on your own. Whatever the manner it ended up in your hands, there's one thing I can guaran-damn-tee you: if you make a habit of using this journal, you'll come out of this journey as a more centered, more fulfilled, and more successful version of yourself.

Despite what you might've heard before, gratitude is not an attitude—it's a practice. This journal is your most powerful tool for making this practice part of your life. And trust me when I tell you: you'll be a better man because of it.

. . . .

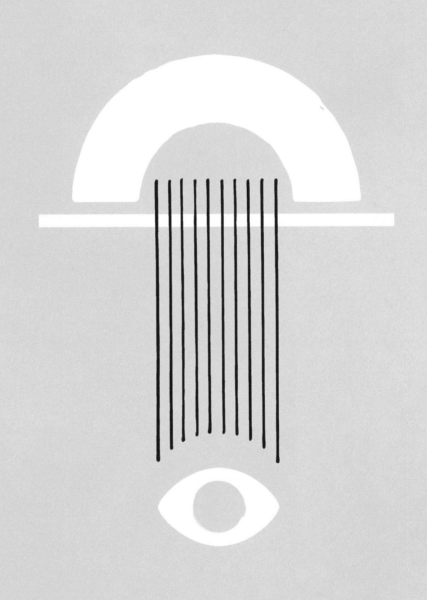

Part 1

AWARENESS

"Acknowledging the good that you already have in your life is the foundation for all abundance."

— Eckhart Tolle, Author

Welcome to the first phase of this gratitude journal.

This book is not going to turn your life around overnight. It's not a magic pill that'll make your problems go "poof."

However, although you may not have a magic pill, you do have something magical in your hands. When you pair it with a pen, you can make magic happen as you write.

It's time to embrace and experience the game-changing power of gratitude. Prepare to level up your life, one day at a time.

1. It's biologically impossible to feel stressed and grateful simultaneously. Think of three things to feel grateful for, so that today, if you feel stress, you can stop and think of them.

2. What's one thing you can do to make today great?

1. What's one thing you enjoyed doing today?

2. What's the best thing that happened today?

1. Gratitude is not an attitude—it's a practice. Today, work on cultivating your gratitude practice, starting by feeling intensely grateful for the following three things:

_____

_____

_____

_____

2. What's one thing you can do to make today great?

_____

_____

_____

1. What could you have done to make today even better?

_____

_____

_____

_____

2. What's the best thing that happened today?

_____

_____

_____

_____

1. You are *you*-nique. There's not a single man on the planet who can do exactly what you can do, in exactly the way you do it. That's powerful stuff. What are three unique qualities about yourself that you're grateful for?

_____

_____

_____

_____

2. What's one thing you can do to make today great?

_____

_____

1. Put a positive spin on something not-so-great that happened today:

_____

_____

_____

_____

2. What's the best thing that happened today?

_____

_____

_____

_____

1. The secret to living is giving. What's one thing you are contributing (personally or professionally) to enhance the lives of others?

_____

_____

_____

_____

2. What's one thing you can do to make today great?

_____

_____

_____

1. Thomas Edison said, "Never go to sleep without a request to your subconscious." What's one major goal you want your mind to help you achieve while you sleep?

_____

_____

_____

_____

2. What's the best thing that happened today?

_____

_____

_____

1. Everyone experiences stress from time to time. And some-times, the best thing you can do to minimize the stress you feel is to write about it. Write down one thing you're stressed about below. After you're done, cross it out as if you were "done" with it. Allow yourself to let that stress go. You're too blessed to be stressed.

_____

_____

_____

2. What's one thing you can do to make today great?

_____

_____

1. Positive thinking isn't a magic cure to all your problems, but it's a good start. Positive thinking leads to positive action, which can lead to positive outcomes. What's one negative thought-pattern you need to let go of right now?

_____

_____

What's a positive thought-pattern you can replace it with?

_____

_____

2. What's the best thing that happened today?

_____

_____

SESSION 1: *Breathe*

The purpose of the breathing sessions in Part I is to let go of current distractions and to keep you from ruminating about past problems or future stresses. We'll do this by bringing your awareness to the present moment.

Step 1: Find a quiet place. Take a seat. Set a timer for three minutes.

Step 2: Close your eyes.

Step 3: Breathe in fully through the nose, and out through the mouth. Repeat this pattern until your timer goes off.

Step 4: When you hear the timer, gently open your eyes and exit with gratitude.

1. Your skills pay the bills. What are three skills you've developed that make you particularly proud?

_____

_____

_____

_____

2. What's one thing you can do to make today great?

_____

_____

_____

_____

· ·

1. How did your skills help you today?

_____

_____

_____

_____

2. What's the best thing that happened today?

_____

_____

_____

_____

1. It's impossible to love anyone else unless you first love yourself. Write down three things you love about yourself:

_____

_____

_____

_____

2. What's one thing you can do to make today great?

_____

_____

_____

_____

1. How did writing what you love about yourself affect your day?

_____

_____

_____

_____

2. What's the best thing that happened today?

_____

_____

_____

_____

1. Gratitude is not an attitude—it's a practice. Today, work on cultivating your gratitude practice, starting by feeling intensely grateful for the following three things:

_____

_____

_____

_____

2. What's one thing you can do to make today great?

_____

_____

_____

1. How could you have made today even better?

_____

_____

_____

_____

2. What's the best thing that happened today?

_____

_____

_____

_____

What is one physical item you're grateful to have in your life right now? Take a few minutes to draw it here *(don't worry, it doesn't have to be fancy)*:

1. When you face your fears, they become smaller. What's one fear you're willing to confront today?

_____

_____

_____

_____

2. What's one thing you can do to make today great?

_____

_____

_____

_____

1. How did you handle coming face-to-face with your fear today?

_____

_____

_____

_____

2. What's the best thing that happened today?

_____

_____

_____

_____

1. The Latin root of the word *decision* literally means "to cut off." Making decisions is about cutting off other possibilities. And that's a good thing, because once you make a definite decision about something you want, you've liberated yourself to pursue that—and only that. Today, make the decision to:

2. What's one thing you can do to make today great?

1. Feeling grateful can improve your overall decision-making. How can you apply gratitude to the decision you made this morning?

2. What's the best thing that happened today?

1. Making and maintaining promises—to yourself and others—helps you grow. It grows your integrity, your confidence, and your sense of self-worth. Promise that today, you will:

_____

_____

_____

_____

2. What's one thing you can do to make today great?

_____

_____

_____

_____

1. Did you keep your promise today? Circle one: **YES   NO**

   How does your answer make you feel?

_____

_____

_____

_____

2. What's the best thing that happened today?

_____

_____

_____

_____

1. Your *self-talk* determines your *self-worth*. Successful self-talk leads to a successful sense of self-worth. What is a one-sentence phrase you can repeat to yourself throughout the day?

_____

_____

_____

_____

2. What's one thing you can do to make today great?

_____

_____

_____

_____

. . . .

1. Today was a success because:

_____

_____

_____

_____

2. What's the best thing that happened today?

_____

_____

_____

_____

1. Sometimes you may take the simplest things for granted: Running water. Electricity. Food. A brain to help you think, dream, and plan for the future. What are three things you've taken for granted in the past but feel genuine gratitude for when you stop to reflect upon them?

_____

_____

_____

_____

2. What's one thing you can do to make today great?

_____

_____

_____

1. What makes you feel loved, and why?

_____

_____

_____

_____

2. What's the best thing that happened today?

_____

_____

_____

_____

1. The past does not equal the future. What's one thing from your past that's holding you back that you must let go of in order to achieve your goals?

_____

_____

_____

_____

2. What's one thing you can do to make today great?

_____

_____

_____

_____

1. What motivated you today?

_____

_____

_____

_____

2. What's the best thing that happened today?

_____

_____

_____

_____

1. Who do you love most in your life?

_____
_____
_____
_____

2. What's one thing you can do to make today great?

_____
_____
_____
_____

1. Who did you interact with today that you want to send a silent "thank you" to?

_____
_____
_____
_____

2. What's the best thing that happened today?

_____
_____
_____
_____

1. List three things you love about the work you do:

_____

_____

_____

_____

2. What's one thing you can do to make today great?

_____

_____

_____

_____

1. What did you accomplish at work today that you're
    proud of?

_____

_____

_____

_____

2. What's the best thing that happened today?

_____

_____

_____

_____

1. Name one of the things in your life that fulfills you the most:

_____

_____

_____

_____

2. What's one thing you can do to make today great?

_____

_____

_____

_____

1. What's one thing you did today that was particularly meaningful?

_____

_____

_____

_____

2. What's the best thing that happened today?

_____

_____

_____

_____

Draw the first thing that pops into your head when you think of the word *grateful.*

1. The powerful thing about questions is that they send you on a quest (read: *quest*-ion). Poor questions lead to poor answers. Great questions lead to great answers.
Poor question: "Why can't I make more money?"
Great question: "What can I do to make more money?"
What's a great question you can ask yourself today?

_____

_____

_____

2. What's one thing you can do to make today great?

_____

_____

_____

1. What's one thing about your life that you're thankful for in this moment?

_____

_____

_____

2. What's the best thing that happened today?

_____

_____

_____

1. Making and maintaining promises—to yourself and others—helps you grow. It grows your integrity, your confidence, and your sense of self-worth.
    Promise that today, you will do the following:

    _____

    _____

    _____

2. What's one thing you can do to make today great?

    _____

    _____

    _____

1. Did you keep your promise to yourself today?
*   **If Yes,** how does that make you feel?
*   **If No,** what can you do to work toward remembering and honoring your promises?

    _____

    _____

    _____

    _____

2. What's the best thing that happened today?

    _____

    _____

    _____

1. What are your top three goals for today?

_____

_____

_____

_____

2. What's one thing you can do to make today great?

_____

_____

_____

1. Did you achieve any of your goals for today?

- **If Yes,** how does that make you feel?
- **If No,** what can you do differently in the future to ensure that you achieve them?

_____

_____

_____

_____

2. What's the best thing that happened today?

_____

_____

_____

S M T W T F S   /   /

1. Name at least one quality you love most about yourself, and why:

_____

_____

_____

_____

2. What's one thing you can do to make today great?

_____

_____

_____

_____

1. What are you looking forward to for tomorrow?

_____

_____

_____

_____

2. What's the best thing that happened today?

_____

_____

_____

_____

1. Success is about doing several small and simple things daily. That's a habit. Describe one of the most useful habits you've developed.

_____

_____

_____

_____

2. What's one thing you can do to make today great?

_____

_____

_____

_____

1. Today, be glad that you:

_____

_____

_____

_____

2. What's the best thing that happened today?

_____

_____

_____

_____

SESSION 2: *Be Like Water*

Step 1: Find a quiet place. Take a seat. Set a timer for five minutes.

Step 2: Close your eyes.

Step 3: Begin by breathing in fully through the nose, and out through the mouth. Become more fully present with your body by focusing on every part of your body, one part at a time, as if it is slowly becoming covered with water. Repeat this pattern until your timer goes off.

Step 4: When you hear the timer, gently open your eyes and exit with gratitude.

1. You can have everything in life you want if you will just help enough other people get what they want.
    What's at least one way you will help others today?

_____

_____

_____

_____

2. What's one thing you can do to make today great?

_____

_____

_____

_____

1. Thomas Edison said, "Never go to sleep without a request to your subconscious." What's one major goal you want your mind to help you achieve while you sleep?

_____

_____

_____

_____

2. What's the best thing that happened today?

_____

_____

_____

1. Complaining gets you nowhere. Refrain from complaining about anything today by going on a "No Complaints Diet." No complaints. All day. Today, every time you have the impulse to complain about something, stop yourself by thinking of something you're grateful for.
    Write three things you're grateful for in your life right now:

    _____

    _____

    _____

    _____

2. What's one thing you can do to make today great?

    _____

    _____

    _____

1. How did your "No Complaints Diet" go today? Could you do it for an entire week?

    _____

    _____

    _____

    _____

2. What's the best thing that happened today?

    _____

    _____

    _____

1. The first thing you do when you're born is breathe. The last
    thing you do before you die is breathe. So, if breathing is the
    first thing you do, and the last thing you do, wouldn't it make
    sense to pay attention to it a bit more?
    Today, I'm grateful for the oxygen that fills my lungs because:

_____

_____

_____

_____

2. What's one thing you can do to make today great?

_____

_____

_____

1. What made you feel powerful today?

_____

_____

_____

_____

2. What's the best thing that happened today?

_____

_____

_____

_____

1. Nothing can prevent a man with a purpose from staying on his path. What is your purpose in life?

_____

_____

_____

_____

2. What's one thing I can do to make today great?

_____

_____

_____

_____

1. Your purpose gives you meaning. Explain what makes you grateful for your life's purpose.

_____

_____

_____

_____

2. What's the best thing that happened today?

_____

_____

_____

_____

1. It's biologically impossible to feel stressed and grateful simultaneously. Today, if you feel stress, stop and think of the following three things to feel grateful for:

_____

_____

_____

_____

2. What's one thing you can do to make today great?

_____

_____

_____

_____

1. What emotion came up today that you are grateful for?

_____

_____

_____

_____

2. What's the best thing that happened today?

_____

_____

_____

_____

1. Making and maintaining promises—to yourself and others—helps you grow. It grows your integrity, your confidence, and your sense of self-worth.
   Promise that today, you will . . .

   _____

   _____

   _____

2. What's one thing you can do to make today great?

   _____

   _____

   _____

1. Did you keep your promise to yourself today?
   - **If Yes,** how does that make you feel?
   - **If No,** what can you do to work toward remembering and honoring your promises?

   _____

   _____

   _____

2. What's the best thing that happened today?

   _____

   _____

   _____

1. Starting each day with an intention will set a positive tone for the entire day. What is your intention for today?

_____

_____

_____

_____

2. What's one thing you can do to make today great?

_____

_____

_____

_____

1. Thomas Edison said, "Never go to sleep without a request to your subconscious." What's one major goal you want your mind to help you achieve while you sleep?

_____

_____

_____

_____

2. What's the best thing that happened today?

_____

_____

_____

1. List your top three goals for today:

_____

_____

_____

_____

2. What's one thing you can do to make today great?

_____

_____

_____

_____

1. Did you achieve any of your goals for today?
- **If Yes,** how does that make you feel?
- **If No,** what can you do differently in the future to ensure that you achieve them?

_____

_____

_____

_____

2. What's the best thing that happened today?

_____

_____

_____

A Time to *Reflect*

As you round out the final corner of your first 30 days, I want to take a moment to congratulate you.
(Cue fist pumps and high fives.)
   I also want to remind you that improving your mental health and developing a positive outlook on the life you lead is no easy task—it takes work. But the work is worth it. Believe that.

But for now, take a moment to reflect upon your first 30 days: How'd it make you feel?

_____

_____

_____

_____

_____

_____

_____

How are you doing physically, mentally, emotionally, and spiritually now that you're 30 days into your new journaling habit?

_____

_____

_____

_____

_____

_____

_____

F·E·E·L·I·N·G·S

Most men bury their emotions. But pretending they don't exist doesn't make them go away. It's like living next to an active volcano, long overdue for an eruption—it's going to erupt eventually. The longer you wait, the more damage it'll cause.

As a man, you need to understand and embrace a very simple truth: It's okay to feel your feelings. Being sad is healthy. Feeling joy is healthy. Crying (gasp) is healthy.

It's even healthy to feel angry. That's right, it can be useful to allow yourself to feel anger or other negative emotions. But it's not useful to be reactive about it. Why? Because reactions can lead to blowups or behaviors you may regret in retrospect.

Replace reactions with responses.

Responsiveness = Thoughtful action

Reactiveness = Immediate and emotional (think: knee-jerk) reactions

Responsiveness is where you want to be. To practice, give yourself a blink of a pause to think about what you're about to do or say prior to expressing your emotions—anger or other-wise. That brief pause gives you a moment to decide whether what you're about to do is going to help you or hurt you.

Bottom line: Embrace the full range of human emotion, responsibly—you'll be a better man because of it.

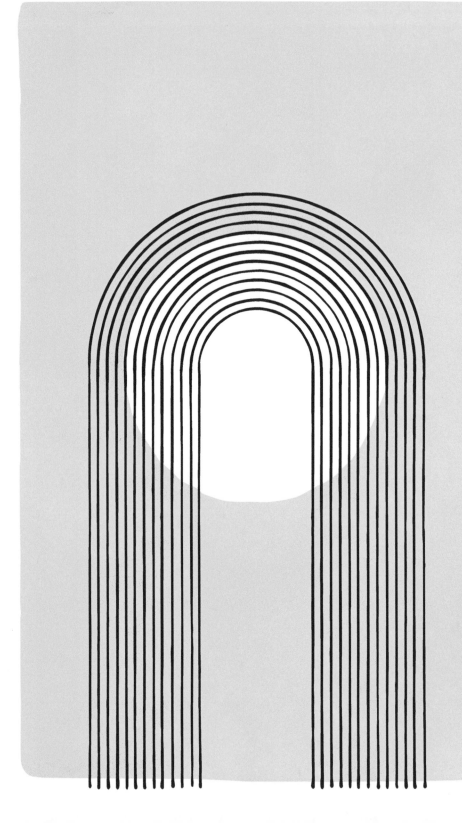

Part II

INTENTION

"At all times and under all circumstances, we have the power to transform the quality of our lives."

— Werner Erhard, Author

Welcome to the second phase of gratitude journaling.

First and foremost, I believe some congratulations are in order. You've successfully cranked out your first 30 days of journaling!

The first phase was all about becoming aware with yourself as a man, exploring your emotions, and learning about the importance of practicing gratitude.

As you move into the next 30 days, you're going to get a bit more intentional and purposeful about your gratitude practice. Part of that will be implementing **Reverse-Gratitude.**

Here's How It *Works* :

Your unconscious mind cannot tell the difference between dreams and reality. So, the faster you can convince your mind to begin feeling grateful for something—even if you don't have it yet—the faster it'll look for ways to help you make it real.

You'll be encouraged to write down something you want—but don't yet have—as if you were *already* grateful for having it.

For example:

- *I'm grateful for being in a healthy relationship.*

- *I'm grateful for having my dream career.*

- *I'm grateful for being in the best shape of my life.*

Don't worry if you can't always think of something new—the point is to put energy toward thinking about and manifesting the things that really matter to you.

My goal for you in the next section is to start feeling a deep and genuine sense of gratitude—physically, mentally, emotionally, and spiritually.

Let's dive in.

1. What does *gratitude* mean to you?

_____

_____

_____

_____

2. *Reverse-Gratitude:* Write down something you want—but
   don't yet have—as if you were *already* grateful for having it.

_____

_____

_____

_____

1. What did you do to feel grateful today?

_____

_____

_____

_____

2. What are you deeply grateful for right now?

_____

_____

_____

_____

1. What are you happy about right now?

_____

_____

_____

_____

2. *Reverse-Gratitude:* Write down something you want—but don't yet have—as if you were already grateful for having it.

_____

_____

_____

_____

1. Think of something you want to happen tomorrow. Write it down and let it sink into your subconscious as you sleep:

_____

_____

_____

_____

2. What are you deeply grateful for right now?

_____

_____

_____

_____

1. There are three things under every man's control:
   • **What he *THINKS*** • **What he *SAYS*** • **What he *DOES***
   How can you be more intentional about each of these today?

_____
_____
_____
_____

2. *Reverse-Gratitude:* Write down something you want—but don't yet have—as if you were already grateful for having it.

_____
_____
_____
_____

1. Who did you connect with today?

_____
_____
_____
_____

2. What are you deeply grateful for right now?

_____
_____
_____
_____

SESSION 1: *Energize + Revitalize*

The purpose of this breathing session is to increase your energy and vitality. This is an energizing breathing session, which means you'll be breathing at a slightly rapid rate. Note: this breathing session should only be done in the morning.

Step 1: Find a comfortable and quiet place. Take a seat. Set a timer for five minutes.

Step 2: Close your eyes.

Step 3: Begin by inhaling (breathing in through the nose) four times rapidly, immediately followed by exhaling (breathing out through the mouth) four times rapidly. Repeat this pattern until your timer goes off.

Step 4: When you hear the timer, gently open your eyes and welcome the day with gratitude.

1. What is your intention for today?

_____
_____
_____
_____

2. *Reverse-Gratitude:* Write down something you want—but don't yet have—as if you were already grateful for having it.

_____
_____
_____
_____

1. What is your intention for tomorrow?

_____
_____
_____
_____

2. What are you deeply grateful for right now?

_____
_____
_____
_____

1. Sharing how you feel about those you love plays a crucial role in your sense of well-being. Who can you share your feelings with today, and what makes this person important to you?

_____
_____
_____
_____

2. *Reverse-Gratitude:* Write down something you want—but don't yet have—as if you were already grateful for having it.

_____
_____
_____

1. How were your feelings received by the person you shared them with today?

_____
_____
_____
_____

2. What are you deeply grateful for right now?

_____
_____
_____

1. Your *self-talk* determines your *self-worth*. What are three self-empowering things you intend on saying to yourself throughout the day?

_____

_____

_____

_____

2. *Reverse-Gratitude:* Write down something you want—but don't yet have—as if you were already grateful for having it.

_____

_____

_____

1. How could you have made today even better?

_____

_____

_____

_____

2. What are you deeply grateful for right now?

_____

_____

_____

_____

1. What are your top three most important outcomes for today?

_____

_____

_____

_____

2. *Reverse-Gratitude:* Write down something you want—but don't yet have—as if you were already grateful for having it.

_____

_____

_____

_____

1. What positive change could you commit to for tomorrow?

_____

_____

_____

_____

2. What are you deeply grateful for right now?

_____

_____

_____

_____

If you could draw a line graph to illustrate your emotions over the past 10 days, what would it look like? Doodle your emotional ups and downs of the past week and a half.

1. Your **WHY** is the most effective possible way in which to articulate your purpose—both to others and yourself. For example, my **WHY** is: "To inspire people everywhere so that they can improve their lives and achieve their goals." What are your "whys"? Use the example above to draft **WHY** statements of your own.

    _____

    _____

    _____

2. *Reverse-Gratitude:* Write down something you want—but don't yet have—as if you were already grateful for having it.

    _____

    _____

    _____

1. How can you better live in alignment with your **WHY**?

    _____

    _____

    _____

2. What are you deeply grateful for right now?

    _____

    _____

    _____

1. What is your intention for today?

_____
_____
_____
_____

2. *Reverse-Gratitude:* Write down something you want—but don't yet have—as if you were already grateful for having it.

_____
_____
_____
_____

. . . .

1. What's your intention for tomorrow?

_____
_____
_____
_____

2. What are you deeply grateful for right now?

_____
_____
_____
_____

1.   There are three things under every man's control:
     • **What he *THINKS***   • **What he *SAYS***   • **What he *DOES***
     How can you be more intentional about each of these today?

_____

_____

_____

_____

2.   *Reverse-Gratitude:* Write down something you want—but
     don't yet have—as if you were already grateful for having it.

_____

_____

_____

_____

1.   How could you have made today even better?

_____

_____

_____

_____

2.   What are you deeply grateful for right now?

_____

_____

_____

_____

S M T W T F S   /   /

1. What are you grateful for in nature, and why?

_____
_____
_____
_____

2. *Reverse-Gratitude:* Write down something you want—but don't yet have—as if you were already grateful for having it.

_____
_____
_____
_____

1. What's one thing you cannot live without, and why?

_____
_____
_____
_____

2. What are you deeply grateful for right now?

_____
_____
_____
_____

1. What do you intend on doing today that will improve your life in the future?

    _____

    _____

    _____

2. *Reverse-Gratitude:* Write down something you want—but don't yet have—as if you were already grateful for having it.

    _____

    _____

    _____

    _____

1. How great does it feel to be you? Write down three positive qualities about yourself below. After you've written them down, take a moment to reflect upon how it makes you feel to think about your own positive attributes. Sit with those feelings.

    _____

    _____

    _____

    _____

2. What are you deeply grateful for right now?

    _____

    _____

    _____

1. What is your greatest strength? How do you intend to use it today?

_____
_____
_____
_____

2. *Reverse-Gratitude:* Write down something you want—but don't yet have—as if you were already grateful for having it.

_____
_____
_____

1. How could you have made today even better?

_____
_____
_____
_____

2. What are you deeply grateful for right now?

_____
_____
_____
_____

1. Your *self-talk* determines your *self-worth*. What are three self-empowering things you intend on saying to yourself throughout the day?

_____

_____

_____

_____

2. *Reverse-Gratitude:* Write down something you want—but don't yet have—as if you were already grateful for having it.

_____

_____

_____

1. What's your favorite hobby? Why?

_____

_____

_____

_____

2. What are you deeply grateful for right now?

_____

_____

_____

_____

1. What is your intention today?

_____
_____
_____
_____

2. *Reverse-Gratitude:* Write down something you want—but don't yet have—as if you were already grateful for having it.

_____
_____
_____
_____

1. What makes your soul smile?

_____
_____
_____
_____

2. What are you deeply grateful for right now?

_____
_____
_____
_____

1. What would you do if you knew you could not fail?

_____

_____

_____

_____

2. *Reverse-Gratitude:* Write down something you want—but don't yet have—as if you were already grateful for having it.

_____

_____

_____

_____

1. Where would you be grateful to go on vacation to?

_____

_____

_____

_____

2. What are you deeply grateful for right now?

_____

_____

_____

_____

1.   What's the one big thing you want to accomplish today?

_____

_____

_____

_____

2.   *Reverse-Gratitude:* Write down something you want—but
     don't yet have—as if you were already grateful for having it.

_____

_____

_____

_____

1.   Who do you love? Who loves you?

_____

_____

_____

_____

2.   What are you deeply grateful for right now?

_____

_____

_____

_____

1. Who do you know that's great at expressing gratitude? What is it about them that makes them great at being grateful?

_____
_____
_____
_____

2. *Reverse-Gratitude:* Write down something you want—but don't yet have—as if you were already grateful for having it.

_____
_____
_____
_____

1. How does it feel when someone expresses their gratitude to you?

_____
_____
_____
_____

2. What are you deeply grateful for right now?

_____
_____
_____
_____

1. What's your intention for today?

_____

_____

_____

_____

2. *Reverse-Gratitude:* Write down something you want—but don't yet have—as if you were already grateful for having it.

_____

_____

_____

_____

1. What's your intention for tomorrow?

_____

_____

_____

_____

2. What are you deeply grateful for right now?

_____

_____

_____

_____

1. As a man, you must make it your duty and obligation to embark on a constant and never-ending journey of growth and success—physically, financially, emotionally, and spiritually. Write down one thing you'll do this week to ensure your future growth and/or success in each of the following areas:

- **Physical Health**
- **Emotions/Socializing**
- **Financial/Business/Career**
- **Spirituality**

_____

_____

_____

2. *Reverse-Gratitude:* Write down something you want—but don't yet have—as if you were already grateful for having it.

_____

_____

_____

1. What made you proud today?

_____

_____

_____

2. What are you deeply grateful for right now?

_____

_____

_____

_____

SESSION 2: *Send Love*

The purpose of this breathing exercise is to cultivate your sense of gratitude for other people.

Step 1: Find a comfortable and quiet place. Take a seat. Set a timer for five minutes.

Step 2: Close your eyes and envision someone you care about.

Step 3: As you hold this person's image in your mind, slowly begin to breathe in the following pattern:

- Inhale slowly and deeply as you hold an image of this person in your mind's eye.
- As you exhale, imagine the air that flows out of your lungs is a cloud of love and gratitude being sent to the person you're thinking about.
- Every inhalation brings forth an image of the person in your mind, while every exhale sends a cloud of love and gratitude to the same person.

Step 4: When you hear the timer, gently open your eyes and welcome the day with gratitude.

1. The secret to living is giving, and there are many ways to give. What's one thing you can do to *give* today without expecting anything in return?

_____
_____
_____
_____

2. *Reverse-Gratitude:* Write down something you want—but don't yet have—as if you were already grateful for having it.

_____
_____
_____
_____

1. How did it feel to give today?

_____
_____
_____
_____

2. What are you deeply grateful for right now?

_____
_____
_____
_____

1. Intention is everything. How do you intend on showing up today?

_____

_____

_____

_____

2. *Reverse-Gratitude:* Write down something you want—but don't yet have—as if you were already grateful for having it.

_____

_____

_____

_____

1. How could you have made today even better?

_____

_____

_____

_____

2. What are you deeply grateful for right now?

_____

_____

_____

_____

1. What are you committed to in your life right now?

_____

_____

_____

_____

2. *Reverse-Gratitude:* Write down something you want—but don't yet have—as if you were already grateful for having it.

_____

_____

_____

_____

1. What's most meaningful to you?

_____

_____

_____

_____

2. What are you deeply grateful for right now?

_____

_____

_____

_____

1. Finish this sentence: **"I'm nothing without** _____ **."**
   Explain your answer.

   _____

   _____

   _____

   _____

2. *Reverse-Gratitude:* Write down something you want—but
   don't yet have—as if you were already grateful for having it.

   _____

   _____

   _____

   _____

1. How do you intend to wake up tomorrow morning?

   _____

   _____

   _____

   _____

2. What are you deeply grateful for right now?

   _____

   _____

   _____

   _____

1. Teaching is the greatest form of learning. Who can you inspire and inform today with what you've learned about yourself and the power of gratitude?

_____

_____

_____

2. *Reverse-Gratitude:* Write down something you want—but don't yet have—as if you were already grateful for having it.

_____

_____

_____

_____

1. What's the biggest problem on your mind right now? What are the possible solutions?

_____

_____

_____

_____

2. What are you deeply grateful for right now?

_____

_____

_____

_____

1. What does "success" mean to you?

_____

_____

_____

_____

2. *Reverse-Gratitude:* Write down something you want—but don't yet have—as if you were already grateful for having it.

_____

_____

_____

_____

. . . .

1. What was successful about today? How can you experience more of it?

_____

_____

_____

_____

2. What are you deeply grateful for right now?

_____

_____

_____

_____

1. What inspires you to get up every morning? Why?

_____

_____

_____

_____

2. *Reverse-Gratitude:* Write down something you want—but don't yet have—as if you were already grateful for having it.

_____

_____

_____

_____

1. Paper is a technology that is often taken for granted. What would life be like if you didn't have paper? How does that change your perspective about it?

_____

_____

_____

_____

2. What are you deeply grateful for right now?

_____

_____

_____

_____

1. Think about the last time you challenged yourself mentally.
   - What did you do?
   - How did it make you feel?

2. *Reverse-Gratitude:* Write down something you want—but don't yet have—as if you were already grateful for having it.

1. Which area of your life do you want to grow?

2. What are you deeply grateful for right now?

1. The best way to get love is to give love. Think about
    someone you love. In the space below, write down what
    you love about them.

    _____

    _____

    _____

    _____

2. *Reverse-Gratitude:* Write down something you want—but
    don't yet have—as if you were already grateful for having it.

    _____

    _____

    _____

1. Think of someone who cares about you (a spouse, friend,
    parent, or child). If this person were asked to write down
    three specific reasons why they love you, what do you
    think they'd write?

    _____

    _____

    _____

2. What are you deeply grateful for right now?

    _____

    _____

    _____

    _____

1. What would you like to experience MORE of in your life?

2. *Reverse-Gratitude:* Write down something you want—but don't yet have—as if you were already grateful for having it.

1. What was the most gratifying thing that happened over the last 30 days?

2. What are you deeply grateful for right now?

A Time to *Reflect*

As you close out your second month of daily journaling, pause for a moment and reflect.

Take a moment to journal about the following:

• What are three positive changes you've noticed within your-self over the past 60 days?

_____

_____

_____

_____

_____

_____

_____

• What are three goals (or benefits) you're looking to gain over the next 30 days of daily journaling?

_____

_____

_____

_____

_____

_____

_____

YOU AREN'T YOUR THOUGHTS

Negative thinking is a powerful, painful, and penetrating state of mind. It's also easier to slip into than thinking positively. Negative thoughts and experiences also tend to outweigh their positive counterparts.

Let's say you're having a really phenomenal day. But then your wife/partner says something that gets under your skin. All of a sudden, your positive day has gone to crap.

You're pissed. You're angry. You're feeling all sorts of negative emotions.

Stop and remember this: What you focus on is what you feel.

To break yourself from this cycle of negativity:

1. **Take a deep breath.** This brings you into the present moment.

2. **Ask yourself,** "What can I feel grateful about right now?" This shifts your focus, bringing positive thoughts and emotions back to the forefront of your brain.

3. **Remind yourself of all the positive experiences you had throughout your day.** This shifts your perspective and helps you realize you've got more to be grateful for than you may realize.

4. **Choose to be positive.** Positive thinking is a habit. But so is negative thinking. Here's the secret: You can choose positivity. This doesn't mean to deny reality. It means to choose positivity over negativity.

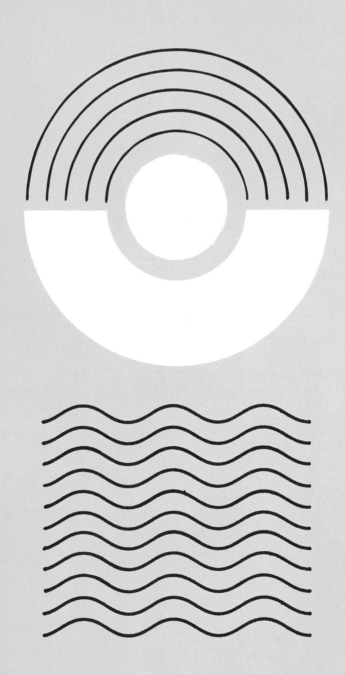

Part III

ACTION

"There is nothing more important to true growth than realizing that you are not the voice of the mind—you are the one who hears it."

— *Michael Singer*, Author/Philosopher

Congratulations! You've completed 60 full days of journaling—that's no easy task! I'd give you a high five and fist bump right about now if we were in the same room.

In Part III, you'll be taking a more personalized and action-oriented approach by beginning each day with a Daily Design.

The *Daily* Design

Over the next 30 days, your first AM prompt will be to conduct a Daily Design, which is a powerful way to set yourself up for success each day.

How It works:

- **Each morning upon rising, write down how you want your day to go** (it helps to keep your journal on your bedside table). What do you want to happen? How do you want to feel? What are the outcomes you're after today?

- **Write your Daily Design as if it's already happened.** For example: I had a great day. I had tons of energy. I made X number of sales today. I really connected with my wife today. I had a phenomenal workout.

Why It's powerful:

- **It forces you to finish your day before it starts.** It puts you in control and gives you a brief moment to think about your day. Want to have a productive day? Write it down. Want to make sure you crush that presentation? Write it down.

Note: **Things don't always go the way you write them out. Don't let that discourage you.** The purpose is to bring your Awareness, Intention, and Actions together to help you stay focused on what you want.

1. *Daily Design:* In the space below, write down exactly how you want your day to go. Remember: Write it down as if it's already happened.

_____

_____

_____

2. *Set Your Top 3 Yearly Goals:* It's goal-setting time. In the space below, write down the three most important things you want to accomplish over the next 12 months.

_____

_____

_____

1. *Magic Moment:* Reflect on something you experienced today that led to a genuine feeling of gratitude or appreciation—a Magic Moment. Write about that experience in the space below. What was your Magic Moment today?

_____

_____

_____

2. With a strong enough **WHY,** any **HOW** is possible. Write down why you want to accomplish each of your Top 3 Yearly Goals. Why are each of these goals important to you?

_____

_____

_____

1. *Daily Design:* In the space below, write down exactly how you want your day to go as if it had already happened.

_____

_____

_____

_____

2. *Set Your Monthly Goal:* Review your Top 3 Yearly Goals and select one goal from your list. Ask yourself, *"What's one thing I need to do within the next 30 days to put me on track to achieve this yearly goal?"* Write your response below. This is your most important goal of the month.

_____

_____

_____

_____

1. What was your Magic Moment today?

_____

_____

_____

2. Below, describe how grateful you'll feel after accomplishing your monthly goal and what it will mean for your future.

_____

_____

_____

_____

1. *Daily Design:* In the space below, write down exactly how you want your day to go.

_____

_____

_____

2. *Set Your Weekly Goal:* Review your Monthly Goal from yesterday and ask yourself, *"What's one thing I need to do within the next seven days to put me on track to achieve my monthly goal?"* Write your response below. This is your most important goal of the week.

_____

_____

_____

1. What was your Magic Moment today?

_____

_____

_____

2. Appreciating your accomplishments is a crucial component of a healthy mindset. It's also something many men don't do enough. What will you do to celebrate and appreciate yourself after you've accomplished your most important goal of the week?

_____

_____

_____

1. *Daily Design:* In the space below, write down exactly how you want your day to go.

_____

_____

_____

_____

2. *Set Your Daily Goal:* Review your Weekly Goal from yester-day and ask yourself, *"What's one thing I need to do today to put me on track to achieve my weekly goal?"* Write your response below. This is your most important goal for today.

_____

_____

_____

_____

1. What was your Magic Moment today?

_____

_____

_____

2. What are three things in your immediate environment (if you're about to sleep, that'd be your bedroom) that you're grateful to have or use?

_____

_____

_____

1. *Daily Design:* In the space below, write down exactly how you want your day to go.

_____

_____

_____

_____

2. What are three actions you're committed to taking or habits you're committed to developing/maintaining in order to live by your definition of success?

_____

_____

_____

_____

. . . .

1. What was your Magic Moment today?

_____

_____

_____

2. What's a habit you'd like to develop? Why?

_____

_____

_____

_____

SESSION 1: *Self*

The purpose of this breathing session is to express appreciation for yourself.

Step 1: Find a comfortable and quiet place. Take a seat. Set a timer for five minutes.

Step 2: Close your eyes and think of all the gratitude and appreciation you've cultivated for yourself over the past few months.

Step 3: Inhale slowly and deeply to the count of five, exhale slowly and deeply to the count of five. Repeat this pattern for the remainder of your session.

Step 4: When you hear the timer, gently open your eyes and exit your session with an expression of gratitude.

1. *Daily Design:* In the space below, write down exactly how you want your day to go.

_____

_____

_____

_____

2. Stress is self-created. What's stressing you out right now, and what is something positive that might come about as a result of this situation?

_____

_____

_____

_____

1. What was your Magic Moment today?

_____

_____

_____

2. In one sentence, describe how you want to feel when you wake up tomorrow morning:

_____

_____

_____

_____

1. *Daily Design:* In the space below, write down exactly how you want your day to go.

_____

_____

_____

_____

2. There are four core areas of life that need your attention if you want to fulfill your potential as a man: **(1) Physical/Financial, (2) Mental, (3) Emotional, and (4) Spiritual.** Write one thing you appreciate about yourself in each of these areas:

_____

_____

_____

_____

1. What was your Magic Moment today?

_____

_____

_____

2. Who will always love you, no matter what? How can you express gratitude to this person?

_____

_____

_____

_____

S   M   T   W   T   F   S   /   /

1. *Daily Design:* In the space below, write down exactly how
    you want your day to go.

    _____
    _____
    _____
    _____

2. If you could write a letter to the younger version of yourself,
    what are three pieces of advice you'd share with him?

    _____
    _____
    _____
    _____

1. What was your Magic Moment today?

    _____
    _____
    _____
    _____

2. What does it mean to live a life of gratitude and
    appreciation?

    _____
    _____
    _____
    _____

Based on the Values prompt (page 109), choose five values you live by and doodle a symbol for each one, along with a corresponding clarifying statement as to why the symbol applies.

1. *Daily Design:* In the space below, write down exactly how you want your day to go.

_____

_____

_____

2. What's most meaningful to you:

   • Personally?

_____

   • Professionally?

_____

_____

1. What was your Magic Moment today?

_____

_____

2. Appreciating your accomplishments is a crucial component of a healthy mindset. It's also something many men don't do enough. Write down one of your recent accomplishments below. What about this accomplishment could you be grateful for?

_____

_____

_____

_____

1. *Daily Design:* In the space below, write down exactly how you want your day to go.

_____

_____

2. After noticing a pattern among countless patients nearing death, a palliative care nurse named Bronnie Ware wrote a book titled *The Top Five Regrets of the Dying,* in which she lays out the following most common regrets people experience on their deathbeds:

   - *I wish I had lived a life true to myself.*
   - *I wish I hadn't worked so hard.*
   - *I wish I'd had the courage to express my feelings.*
   - *I wish I had stayed in touch with my friends.*
   - *I wish that I had let myself be happier.*

- Which of these regrets do you need to appreciate or pay more attention to?

_____

- Which of these regrets are you doing well with already?

_____

1. What was your Magic Moment today?

_____

_____

2. What are your three greatest strengths, and how did you use them today?

_____

_____

1. *Daily Design:* In the space below, write down exactly how you want your day to go.

_____

_____

_____

_____

2. Write one example of how you're living a life true to yourself:

_____

_____

_____

_____

1. What was your Magic Moment today?

_____

_____

_____

_____

2. What's one action you took today that deserves a moment of gratitude or appreciation?

_____

_____

_____

_____

1. *Daily Design:* In the space below, write down exactly how you want your day to go.

_____

_____

_____

2. Hard work plays an integral role in fulfilling your highest potential as a man. But hard work has a limit—and surpassing it leads to burnout, decaying health, and psychological degradation.

    Are you working too hard? Circle: YES NO

    What contributes to that, and what will happen if you continue in this direction?

_____

_____

_____

1. What was your Magic Moment today?

_____

_____

2. In one sentence, describe how you want to feel when you wake up tomorrow morning:

_____

_____

_____

1. *Daily Design:* In the space below, write down exactly how you want your day to go.

_____

_____

_____

_____

2. Write one example of when you had the courage to express your feelings. What was the result?

_____

_____

_____

_____

1. What was your Magic Moment today?

_____

_____

_____

_____

2. How can you express your feelings more often?

_____

_____

_____

_____

SESSION 2: *The Goal*

The purpose of this breathing exercise is to help you connect with—and achieve—your biggest goal. I would suggest practicing this one on a daily basis.

Step 1: Find a comfortable and quiet place. Take a seat. Set a timer for five minutes.

Step 2: Close your eyes and envision yourself achieving your greatest, most ambitious goal. Hold this image in your mind's eye.

Step 3: As you continue to hold the image of yourself achieving your goal in your mind, begin breathing— inhaling and exhaling at a slow and steady pace.

Step 4: With each inhalation, allow the outcome you seek to get more and more detailed.

Step 5: When you hear the timer, release the image and stand and exit your session with confidence, knowing you'll achieve the goal you've envisioned—even if you don't know how yet.

S   M   T   W   T   F   S   /   /

1. *Daily Design:* In the space below, write down exactly how you want your day to go.

_____

_____

_____

_____

2. How are you staying in touch with friends and/or loved ones?

_____

_____

_____

_____

1. What was your Magic Moment today?

_____

_____

_____

_____

2. Who do you need to get in touch with and express your gratitude and appreciation for this week?

_____

_____

_____

_____

1. *Daily Design:* In the space below, write down exactly
    how you want your day to go.

_____

_____

_____

_____

2. Author and motivational speaker Earl Nightingale wrote that
    "Succes is the progressive realization of a worthy goal or
    ideal." What are you doing to bring happiness into your life?

_____

_____

_____

_____

1. What was your Magic Moment today?

_____

_____

_____

2. What's a goal you're working on right now that, though chal-
    lenging, brings you joy and happiness while you work on it?

_____

_____

_____

_____

1. *Daily Design:* In the space below, write down exactly
    how you want your day to go.

    _____

    _____

    _____

    _____

2. Who makes you feel appreciated? How do they show
    you appreciation?

    _____

    _____

    _____

    _____

1. What was your Magic Moment today?

    _____

    _____

    _____

    _____

2. Reflect on the person you noted above, who makes you
    feel appreciated. What are ways you can show your
    appreciation for them?

    _____

    _____

    _____

    _____

GET CREATIVE

Write the words *I'm Grateful For* in the middle of this page and draw a circle around it. Now, create a mind-map of everything you're grateful for in your life.

1. *Daily Design:* In the space below, write down exactly how you want your day to go.

_____

_____

_____

_____

2. What are you looking forward to today?

_____

_____

_____

_____

1. What was your Magic Moment today?

_____

_____

_____

_____

2. What seemingly small change can you make to improve your day tomorrow?

_____

_____

_____

_____

1. *Daily Design:* In the space below, write down exactly how you want your day to go.

_____
_____
_____
_____

2. What's your favorite part of your morning routine?

_____
_____
_____
_____

1. What was your Magic Moment today?

_____
_____
_____
_____

2. What's your favorite part of your evening routine?

_____
_____
_____
_____

1. *Daily Design:* In the space below, write down exactly how you want your day to go.

_____

_____

_____

_____

2. What will you do to show yourself gratitude and appreciation today?

_____

_____

_____

_____

. . . .

1. What was your Magic Moment today?

_____

_____

_____

_____

2. What are your Top 3 habits for cultivating gratitude?

_____

_____

_____

_____

1. *Daily Design:* In the space below, write down exactly how you want your day to go.

_____

_____

_____

2. Mini-habits are small actions you can take, practically any-time, that can have a compounding impact on your life over time. What are three positive mini-habits you've developed (or want to develop) to cultivate a sustained sense of grate-fulness in your daily life?

_____

_____

_____

_____

1. What was your Magic Moment today?

_____

_____

_____

_____

2. Write about a difficult moment you have faced that ended up teaching you a valuable life lesson.

_____

_____

_____

_____

1. *Daily Design:* In the space below, write down exactly how you want your day to go.

_____

_____

_____

_____

2. What do you love about yourself?

_____

_____

_____

_____

· ·

1. What was your Magic Moment today?

_____

_____

_____

_____

2. What matters most to you?

_____

_____

_____

_____

1. *Daily Design:* In the space below, write down exactly how you want your day to go.

_____
_____
_____
_____

2. Doing something you're afraid of is a great way to expand your comfort zone and build your confidence. What's one thing you fear doing that you could try doing today?

_____
_____
_____
_____

1. What was your Magic Moment today?

_____
_____
_____
_____

2. What was the result of doing what you were afraid of today?

_____
_____
_____
_____

1. *Daily Design:* In the space below, write down exactly how you want your day to go.

_____

_____

_____

_____

2. Weather is an underappreciated resource. What can you appreciate about the weather today? Rain or shine, find something to feel grateful for.

_____

_____

_____

_____

1. What was your Magic Moment today?

_____

_____

_____

_____

2. Who do you need to get in touch with and express your gratitude and appreciation for this week?

_____

_____

_____

_____

1. *Daily Design:* In the space below, write down exactly how you want your day to go.

_____
_____
_____
_____

2. One of the keys to living a fulfilling life is to focus on what's most important. Below, write down what's most important to you right now.

_____
_____
_____
_____

1. What was your Magic Moment today?

_____
_____
_____

2. In one sentence, describe how you want to feel when you wake up tomorrow morning:

_____
_____
_____

1. *Daily Design:* In the space below, write down exactly how you want your day to go.

_____

_____

_____

_____

2. Whenever you feel stress, find someone to bless. What can you do today to help someone who needs more than you do?

_____

_____

_____

_____

1. What was your Magic Moment today?

_____

_____

_____

_____

2. Write about a time when someone helped you out. How did it make you feel?

_____

_____

_____

_____

1. *Daily Design:* In the space below, write down exactly how you want your day to go.

_____

_____

_____

_____

2. What do you appreciate about the work you do?

_____

_____

_____

_____

1. What was your Magic Moment today?

_____

_____

_____

_____

2. What brought you genuine joy, gratitude, or happiness today?

_____

_____

_____

_____

1. *Daily Design:* In the space below, write down exactly how you want your day to go.

_____

_____

2. As a man, everything you say and do is a reflection of your values. Clarifying your values gets you closer to living a purposeful, passionate life, bursting with gratitude. In the space below, choose a value, then clarify it with an action-able statement that explains how you'll live it daily.

For example:
- Value: *Integrity*
- Clarifying Statement:

  Always do the right thing, even when no one is watching.

Now write your own below:
- Value:
- Clarifying Statement:

_____

1. What was your Magic Moment today?

_____

_____

_____

2. What could you have done better today?

_____

_____

_____

1. *Daily Design:* In the space below, write down exactly
    how you want your day to go.

    _____
    _____
    _____
    _____

2. Who deserves an expression of appreciation from you today?
    Write their name below, and reach out to them at some point
    today via phone call, text, or email to express your gratitude.

    _____
    _____
    _____
    _____

1. What was your Magic Moment today?

    _____
    _____
    _____
    _____

2. How did the person you expressed your appreciation
    for respond?

    _____
    _____
    _____
    _____

1. *Daily Design:* In the space below, write down exactly how you want your day to go.

_____

_____

_____

2. Boxer Mike Tyson famously said, "Everyone has a plan till they get punched in the mouth." In life, things don't always go as planned. How can you be grateful about finding a different way to achieve your goal next time things don't go how you planned?

_____

_____

_____

1. What was your Magic Moment today?

_____

_____

_____

2. Write down a goal you think might be out of reach for you. Then, write what steps you could potentially take to make it more attainable.

_____

_____

_____

_____

1. *Daily Design:* In the space below, write down exactly how you want your day to go.

_____

_____

_____

2. Emotion comes from motion. You can change or incite new emotional states by moving your body. For example, if you're feeling low on energy, you can jump in the air, clap your hands, and yell "Boom!" to generate energy. In the space below, create a gratitude movement you can execute anytime you feel like your gratitude tank is close to empty.

_____

_____

_____

_____

1. What was your Magic Moment today?

_____

_____

_____

2. What are some things you appreciated most about this journaling experience?

_____

_____

_____

A Time to *Reflect*

Congratulations! You've completed 90 full days of journaling. Use the space below to reflect on your experience:
What did you learn and gain from this experience? Highlight your breakthroughs, Magic Moments, rewards, and any goals you've got moving forward.

_____

_____

_____

_____

_____

_____

_____

_____

_____

_____

_____

_____

_____

_____

_____

_____

_____

_____

_____

_____

_____

_____

THERE'S POWER IN GRATITUDE

There's real power in gratitude. In a series of studies on Gratitude, Robert Emmons, the world's leading scientific expert on the subject, shares the powerful benefits you can gain through the simple practice of gratitude journaling.

After studying more than 1,000 participants between the ages of eight and 80, Emmons reports that people who regularly practice gratitude experience a wide range of benefits by maintaining the habit, including the following:

Physical health: People who practice gratitude regularly have strong immune systems, lower blood pressure, and better sleep. They exercise more, too!

Psychological wellness: People who practice gratitude regularly experience more positive emotions, are more optimistic, and have higher levels of focus and alertness.

Social benefits: People who practice gratitude regularly are more compassionate, forgiving, and outgoing.

The points above are just a few of the benefits people gain from practicing gratitude.

I'm sure by now, you've enjoyed many of these benefits within your own life as well. If you like what you've experienced, continue to cultivate and nurture this habit of gratitude journaling. So don't stop—because gratitude journaling is a habit you can keep up with for the rest of your life.

One Final *Note*

When I teach men about improving their mental health, or when I share the game-changing impact of gratitude journaling, one of the most important points I like to emphasize is this:

These are *habits* that need to be maintained.

If you stop exercising, your muscles shrink, and you lose your strength. Similarly, if you slack on your journaling and stop working on improving your mindset, guess what happens? The journals lose their strength.

Don't let that happen to you. Stay on your game. Keep using the concepts and tools you've equipped yourself with over the past 90 days. Keep growing your mental muscles. Keep cultivating gratitude.

If your life is worth living, it's worth recording. To maintain your momentum, I'd suggest picking up another copy of this journal or buying a blank journal to continue your daily journaling habit.

Be sure to keep your journals after you finish each of them. Over time, you'll build up a collection of books to look back on. It's a beautiful way to maintain a record of your life experiences, your personal development, and your continued growth as a man.

With respect and gratitude,

Dean

RESOURCES

. . . .

The Book of Joy: Lasting Happiness in a Changing World by His Holiness the Dalai Lama, Archbishop Desmond Tutu, and Douglas Carlton Abrams

Why Gratitude Is Good by Robert Emmons:
greatergood.berkeley.edu/article/item/why_gratitude_is_good

Dean Bokhari's Meaningful Show Podcast

- Podcast Homepage: MeaningfulHQ.com
- Apple Podcasts: DeanBokhari.com/go/apple
- Spotify: DeanBokhari.com/go/spotify

REFERENCES

Introduction

Newmark, Amy, and Deborah Norville. *Chicken Soup for the Soul: The Power of Gratitude: 101 Stories about How Being Thankful Can Change Your Life.* United States: Chicken Soup for the Soul, 2016.

Part I: Awareness

Dalai Lama, Desmond Tutu, and Douglas Carelton Adams. *The Book of Joy: Lasting Happiness in a Changing World.* Leicester: Thorpe, Isis, 2018.

Eha, Brian Patrick. "Zig Ziglar and the Importance of Helping Others." *Entrepreneur*, November 30, 2012. https://www.entrepreneur.com/article/225131.

Epicurus. "Epicurus Quotes (Author of *The Art of Happiness*)." Goodreads. Accessed September 25, 2020. https://www.goodreads.com/author/quotes/114041.Epicurus.

Ferriss, Timothy. *Tools of Titans: The Tactics, Routines, and Habits of Billionaires, Icons, and World-Class Performers.* Boston, MA: Houghton Mifflin Harcourt, 2017.

Seneca, Lucius Annaeus. "Seneca (Author of *Letters from a Stoic*)." Goodreads. Accessed September 25, 2020. https://www.goodreads.com/author/show/4918776.Seneca.

Tolle, Eckhart. *A New Earth: Awakening to Your Life's Purpose*. London: Penguin Books, 2018.

UC Davis Health, Public Affairs and Marketing. "Gratitude Is Good Medicine." UC Davis Health, November 25, 2015. https://health.ucdavis.edu/medicalcenter/features/2015-2016/11/20151125_gratitude.html.

Part II: Intention

Interview with William Warren Bartley, cited in Bartley, William Warren *Werner Erhard: The Transformation of a Man: The Founding of est*. New York: Clarkson N. Potter, Inc, 1978.

Haidt, Jonathan. *The Happiness Hypothesis: Putting Ancient Wisdom to the Test of Modern Science*. London: Cornerstone Digital, 2015.

Hill, Napoleon. *Think and Grow Rich: The Original*, an official publication of The Napoleon Hill Foundation. United States: Sound Wisdom, 2019, First Edition 1937.

Singer, Michael A. *The Untethered Soul: The Journey Beyond Yourself*. Oakland, CA: New Harbinger Publications, 2013.

Part III: Action

Deida, David. *The Way of the Superior Man: A Spiritual Guide to Mastering the Challenges of Women, Work, and Sexual Desire*. N.p.: ReadHowYouWant.com, Limited, 2008.

Drucker, Peter. *The Effective Executive*. United Kingdom: Taylor & Francis, 2018. (January 3, 2006).

Emmons, Robert. "Why Gratitude Is Good." Greater Good Magazine. Greater Good Science Center, November 16, 2010. https://greatergood. berkeley.edu/article/item/why_gratitude_is_good.

Erhard, Werner. "The End of Starvation: Creating an Idea Whose Time Has Come." Werner Erhard - The Hunger Project Source Document, 1977. http://www.wernererhard.net/thpsource.html.

"A Quote by Mike Tyson." Goodreads. Goodreads. Accessed September 25, 2020. https://www.goodreads.com/quotes/1194638-everyone-has-a-plan-till-they-get-punched-in-the.

Murray, William Hutchison. *The Scottish Himalayan Expedition*. London: Dent, 1951.

Earl Nightingale Quotes. BrainyQuote.com, BrainyMedia Inc, 2020. https://www.brainyquote.com/quotes/earl_nightingale_383460, accessed December 3, 2020.

Tracy, Brian. *Goals! How to Get Everything You Want—Faster Than You Ever Thought Possible*. Canada: ReadHowYouWant.com, Limited, 2008.

Ware, Bronnie. *The Top Five Regrets of the Dying: A Life Transformed by the Dearly Departing*. Carlsbad, CA: Hay House Inc., 2019.

Contributors to Wikimedia. "Gratitude." Wikiquote. Wikimedia Foundation, Inc., August 26, 2020. https://en.wikiquote.org/wiki/Gratitude.

ACKNOWLEDGMENTS

My mother and father—who were the first to teach me about the power of gratitude. My wife and daughter—life wouldn't be life without you. My brother—you're my best friend. I'm grateful for and love you all.

I'm also grateful to have learned about the power of practicing gratitude journaling from some of the world's greatest thinkers, including Stephen Covey, Tony Robbins, Brené Brown, Simon Sinek, Tim Ferriss, and Jim Rohn.

. . . .

ABOUT THE AUTHOR

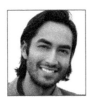 Dean Bokhari is an author, entrepreneur, motivational speaker, and host of the popular self-improvement podcast Dean Bokhari's Meaningful Show. He is sought after internationally as a speaker on habits, productivity, motivation, meaningful work, and leadership. He is the founder of FlashBooks Book Summaries (GetFlashNotes.com), one of the largest nonfiction book summary platforms in the world. His work has been featured in Lifehacker, HuffPost, *Inc., Lifehack,* and *Fast Company,* among others. Dean's mission is to inspire and empower people everywhere to improve their lives and achieve their goals.

Dean Bokhari's Homepage + Personal Development Blog:
* DeanBokhari.com

Dean Bokhari's Meaningful Show Podcast:
* Podcast Homepage: MeaningfulHQ.com
* Apple Podcasts: DeanBokhari.com/go/apple
* Spotify: DeanBokhari.com/go/spotify